I HAVE NO TIME FOR CANCER!

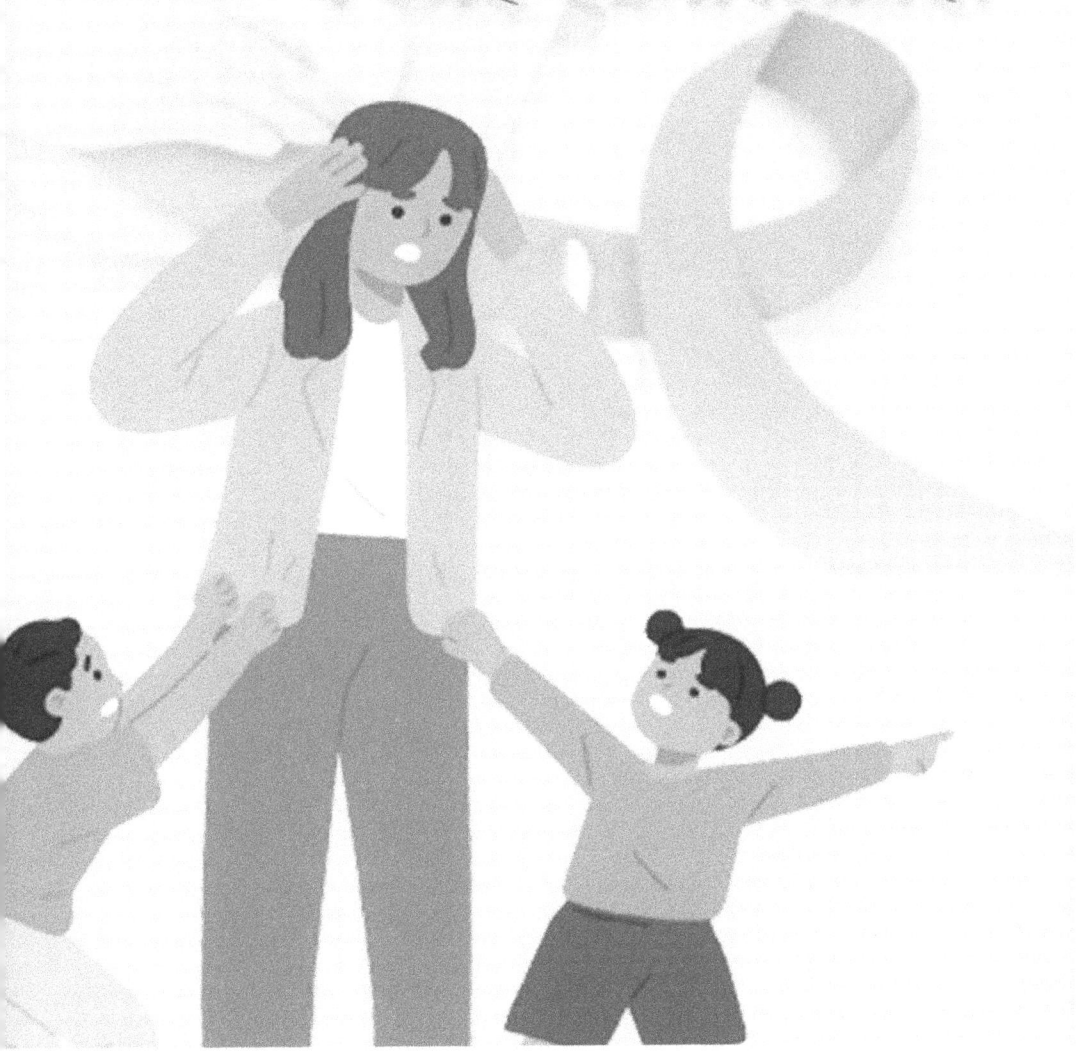

KATHY MOORE

I HAVE
NO TIME
FOR CANCER!

KATHY MOORE

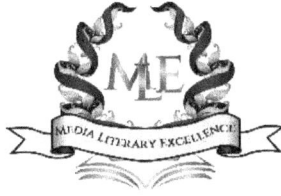

I HAVE NO TIME FOR CANCER!

ISBN (Paperback): 978-1-958082-52-2
ISBN (Ebook): 978-1-958082-53-9

Printed in the United States of America

CONTENTS

FOREWORD

I hope this book brings smiles and some chuckles to those of you out there fighting cancer. Laughter was definitely something I wanted and needed while going through it myself. Boredom and discomfort are not a good combination, and those of you going through treatments know what I mean. Try and make the best of your situation. Everyone's environment is different. As for myself, I'm a single mother. On top of that, any family members I have are a couple of states away. But, I have been blessed to have a great church family that prayed for me and some members that also offered practical help. So, don't be afraid to ask for help when you need it. Also, make sure you're eating healthy (natural/organic foods preferably), hydrating yourself…and, of course, *laughing whenever possible.* Find humor in whatever you can…sitcoms, comedy movies, and enjoyable people to be around. Laughter IS the best medicine. Perhaps you will at least find my bad luck entertaining.

CHAPTER 1

Toward the end of 2016 my friend and church mate of a couple of years did my mammography, as usual. In fact, we met over my boobs. She's a great x- ray technician. With this particular mammogram, the radiologist was concerned with my 3D x-rays, which was also confirmed by the doctor who would become my surgeon.

When I had my appointment with the surgeon and she reviewed my pathology report with me, I was informed that it looked to only be around .8 or .9cm. I was to come in for a biopsy not too much later. It was a painful ordeal, but, a quick procedure. I'm not sure, but, I believe I came back in another day to have measurements taken of the tumor. The equipment being very modern, they could get the exact measurements of where the tumor was to be surgically removed, and with margins. Seemed ok so far...

On my next visit to my surgeon, however, I came to find out that the tumorwas in fact .9cms, but, that it was HER2+ (which in quasi non-medical terms, is the more aggressive type due to a protein). My surgeon did have a good bedside manner, but she couldn't put a positive spin on this really. The plan was targeted radiation and chemo. (I rarely ever say "chemotherapy" as I find nothing therapeutic about it). This wasn't a good day to have to go to work afterwards…but, I did. However, I made a stop at Dunkin Donuts, for some comfort first. I think crying into my croissant in their parking lot was the only time I cried, but, not for long. I'm a practical planner, so this definitely upset my apple cart. With two boys, ages 11 and 13, a mortgage, and a host of other bills, I was concerned.

CHAPTER 2

One good thing about having connections (my x-ray friend) is getting a quick surgery date. I believe three or so weeks later I was tattooed and on the operating table. I was cut in three places: one for the tumor, another for a couple of lymph nodes to be tested, and the third for the radiation device which resembled an egg beater. The surgery went fine, and so did the short time in recovery. A friend of mine's husband picked me up from the hospital and let me stay at their home for a couple of days to recover. My ex-husband stayed with the boys.

I don't recall the exact details of this egg-beater looking thing that sat inside by boob sideways, but, I didn't like it. It was in me for about a week and stuck out of me a little. I felt like a tea pot with a spout. Feeling it and changing gauze was not so fun.

When I went to the radiation doctor to review the treatment, he determined it could not be done – *I was too leaky*. So, the next to-do was to heal and then visit the oncologist. There were many things being said to me, and papers (many papers in a binder) and all I remember during that appointment was saying to the doctor and nurse "Oh my God, I don't have TIME for this!" (meaning, the treatment plan). Oh, and I can't forget them mentioning that the lady before me walked out – and she only needed radiation!

CHAPTER 3

I realized that I was a baby when on my first chemo day; the friend who dropped me off at the hospital and was going to pick me up didn't come into the hospital with me. Well, okay… "bye". I was a little nervous. However, after being there a while, I realized how nice the nurses were, there was TV, and I knew they would serve me lunch, so, how bad could it be? I remember asking the nurse toward the end if I could drive myself to and fro and she said "Yes. It's two or three days later that you might not be feeling so good". And, she was right. I had forgotten to have the anti-nausea medication filled beforehand that my oncologist had given me, and, so, there I was two, three, and four days later throwing up off and on… whether I ate or not. I did not make that mistake again; however, the medication didn't work that well anyway. One of the drugs, called Adriamycin, nicknamed "the red devil", was the cause of that. …Bad devil, bad.

After the first two sessions, or so, I noticed there was a side effect pattern, so I was able to predict what I was able to do – from working, to errand- running, to cleaning and laundry. I was only able to work 35% of the time (by the grace of God, my employer was okay with this), did my food shopping on my best day, and as far as cleaning, I had to have a friend who cleans part time for a living come every couple of weeks. I couldn't fathom cleaning bathrooms or vacuuming the carpets with how I felt. Now, 80% bald, I think I scored some baldness points. My younger son helped with the laundry and dishwasher. And, when my ex-husband came by to check on me and the boys he would take out the trash and clean up a bit. My boys aren't the neatest.

During this first cycle (not session), which was every two weeks for three months, the company I was working for shut down...and without notice to its employees. So, this bald, single parent who looked like a rooster and who couldn't work all the time between being sick or having appointments needed to find a new job. Ha, ha, ha.

First, I filed for unemployment. Second, I updated my resume. And third, I asked for help from the nurse navigator from the hospital, who I was told would help me in any way she could. With her help, we submitted several charitable applications, and by the grace of God, three did help and in a month's time, I had some financial assistance. Unemployment was coming in also. So, my bill payments were not always on time, but, I was "getting by".

During these months, my church family was praying for me. I was making it to church about half the time. A lot of people thought that was a good sign, but, they didn't see me on the first week of my chemo treatments, only the second. Some even made a meal for me and my boys. One friend made spaghetti and meatballs thinking the boys would like that. Little did I know, they wouldn't like the different tomato sauce. And this was a big tray of it, so, I had to eat it all a little at a time. In addition, tomato sauce and spicy foods were on You Should Avoid list, but I didn't want my friend's time and energy to go to waste. Another friend invited me to her home. Since I was frightening the first week after chemo, I only let people see me the second. So, it was bad week, good week, bad week, good week. My body was in pain. It seemed to feel like a combination of the flu and morning sickness… with delirium thrown in. Although some people wanted to visit, I was too stinky, I thought. The chemicals that you sweat out don't smell like roses, either. Showering was painful some days. It hurt to lift my hands to my head. However, on my good weeks, I got to see my church peeps on Sunday, cowgirl hat on and a smile on my face. I came to realize that some seemed to want me to wear a wig. But, I was not having that. It seemed that the ladies were concerned that my baldness would affect me I think. I thought, not so much. If they only knew how I felt physically, they'd know that I didn't care so much about that.

So, it was many microwavable dinners, ordering in at times, and letting one of my sons experiment in the kitchen a little. Job searching was every weekday that I got out of the house. I went to the library and I eventually drove around handing out resumes as my hair started growing in a little. I applied to jobs I thought I was qualified for, but also may have flexibility in the hours. It wasn't looking good.

It was around this time that I developed a very painful urinary tract infection. Not only that, but, it didn't go away after the first round of antibiotics. I needed two. It was a six week ordeal. God was really testing my patience. My immune system was really being challenged.

CHAPTER 4

I was in my second cycle of treatments. They were getting easier with a different group of chemicals, but, now they were weekly. My body was getting tired from the whole enchilada. I always had a terrible taste in my mouth, nothing from food to water tasted right, and my vision was blurred, which I didn't like at all, because I wanted to read books. The eyes were still good enough for driving though. It was summertime and I took my younger son on errands, shopping, library, etc. He was my companion. The trouble with being out in public or driving was my diarrhea issue. I did have it for months at this point, but, now I was trying to get out more, even hand out resumes on occasion, and also take my son out for lunch sometimes. So, if I ate that day, and I was in a store, etc., I would be running to the restroom without much forewarning. I tried wearing a diaper, but realized early on that it didn't work. I would blow them out. At this point, I was getting a few interviews, but, they weren't for me, or I wasn't for them. There was one I had interest in, however, but, he said in a roundabout way that when my treatments were done to contact him again and see if he's hiring.

Worn out and discouraged, I told my oncologist during a follow up appointment that I am having trouble finding new employment. He offered to write me up a note that I am okay to work, but, I knew that that wasn't going to work. My interviewers were of course interviewing people without wraps on their heads or that needed flexibility for medical appointments like me. I just continued to apply to more jobs.

I also set up an I Can Taste Food Again restaurant gathering with my church family after service one Sunday. I was free from everything tasting like chemicals…and I couldn't wait to have my first meal be a nice juicy steak. Almost the whole congregation joined me for my exciting meal and companionship. We couldn't get a giant table, but we were close in spirit.

CHAPTER 5

After 3 weeks of a break, it was now radiation time. The doctor wanted to allow 5 or 6 weeks and I said "No, no, let's get the ball rolling here; I have to get a job soon". In fact, my unemployment would be running out in a month or so.

During week two of radiation, I had developed a yeast infection... coincidentally, under the breast that was being treated. The radiation wasn't the cause per say, but, not wearing a bra much did. There's that immune system again! This made the urinary tract infection that I had seem like child's play. I had all these ointments to put on, and it took three or four weeks until it was gone...all the while, my breast was getting slow sunburn. And, each weekday I drove up to the hospital for six weeks for my radiation, minus two days to recuperate when the infection was bad. But, red, itchy, and burned boob made it! This was a milestone for me. This would be the end to two treatments, with only immunotherapy remaining. Whoo-hooo!

Immunotherapy, which I finished about two months ago, was just one chemical. It went on for several months every three weeks, but side effects weren't bad. Probably the most annoying, were the heart palpitations that it gave me. It is known to be a little hard on the heart. One needs to even have aheart scan every other month to make sure it's pumping on course. But, naturally, with my luck, it had slowed down my pumping a little, so they had to stop the therapy for a while until it regained its normal pace...and then they resumed. I was also advised to go to my primary care physician who put me on a mild dose of high blood pressure medication and scheduled me for a visit to the cardiologist. Since I've had a mild case of mitral valve prolapse for years, the immunotherapy drug was exacerbating it a bit. However, the cardiologist did a couple of tests and my heart appeared to be okay. I justneed to follow up every so often.

At this point, job-wise, I've gone on several interviews, and considered them practice at the time. But, I knew that I was getting closer to my goal. My hair was almost presentable too. I had more confidence and that brought more job searching.

Then I got the call...

While at the library one late morning I received a call from the owner of a company who said, he got my resume from one of his employees from a recent drop-off. And, while I had done some drop-offs, I didn't recall this one. We had a 40-minute conversation, he in his car, and me in the library lobby. Honestly, I couldn't understand 40% of what he was saying because of my stupid phone that gets lousy reception. However, I didn't want to blow this phone interview, so I let him do most of the talking and

I caught enough to get by. He had just fired the woman he had at one of his locations and needed someone to start training right away. He made his pitch, as he called it, and I was sold. He also let me enjoy my Thanksgiving weekend that was coming up first. All excited, and mentioning this to my ex-husband, he said, "That was me!"

So, it turned out that when I had given some to him two weeks prior that he ended up giving one to that "employee". That employee knew that they were hiring for another location.

The beauty of the job…

I actually found (or it found me) a job in which I would be off on Wednesdays. And, what did I need? A job that I could go to the hospital and get my infusion during a weekday for a couple of hrs. God made a way for me, ahhhh.

CHAPTER 6

Good-bye cowgirl hat…

At this point, I stopped wearing my hat/bandana combo. Although I'm a native New Yorker, I liked the cowgirl hat – it became part of me too. Thinking back, the interesting thing about the hair loss was that the people I knew cared more about that than *I did*. How I felt physically overshadowed that big time. And, I hated the idea of a wig. That seemed icky to me. Just so, you know, I didn't wear my cowgirl hat on any interviews. I used one of those wrap things. It wasn't me, but served its purpose.

So, during my time at my new job, my side effects have faded away…some faster than others. My memory has improved (only a little chemo-brain as it's called), along with my vision, my energy, nausea, bad taste in my mouth, diarrhea, heart palpitations. I'm a month and a half out from my last immunotherapy infusion, which brought on palpitations. But, now that that last drug administered is out of my system, I am falling asleep easier and doing more with my days…I started this book, I'm doing some little home improvements to prepare my house for sale next year, and I joined a gym.

I can reflect now, and find humor in a lot of it. Things that really weren't funny at the time. I'll never forget my younger son doing his first load of laundry and had used bleach instead of detergent. He thought it did the same thing. Therefore, some things had to be thrown out, some things we kept and stand as a reminder of how silly things can be.

The only drug I am on now is my post-cancer pill, which I will have to take every day for five or ten years (still to be determined). The two potential side effects are joint pain and hot flashes. I have number two, and it feels like menopause again. If I'm going to sweat, I rather it be by exercising! I am doing well with the working out though. I have to get rid of the weight I gained after chemo and from my desk job.

Another thing I'd like to get rid of is "Portia", my chemo port. The nurses told me at my last immunotherapy appointment that it normally stays in for a year. It doesn't bother me physically, but it's the psychological aspect of it that bothers me. They mentioned that it is precautionary and also makes it easier if I were to need blood drawn, but, said that when I see the doctor next time to inquire about its removal. When the port is out, I will truly feel finished and enjoy making time for everything else but cancer.

I hope we know the cure for cancer soon and how to prevent it. There is information out there. One's pH has to be alkaline. Cancer can't grow in an alkaline environment. Do the research. I personally use lemon juice in my glasses of water, and I eat a couple of apricot seeds per day. If you're the one battling cancer, do not go around saying "I have cancer". You are what you think! And, don't lie in bed all day if you can help it! Certainly, get your rest…but if you are able go to work, work. If you can drive safely, do your errands. You'll realize how strong you really are. If you are not this lucky, have people that care about you take you to and from your treatments, have them visit you and bring you what you need, engage in conversation with them (in or out of pajamas!), and watch funny shows on TV. And, if you are the family member of someone battling cancer, ask him or what he or she needs, help him or her with whatever that is, pray for him or her, and give that person, your loved one, a reason to laugh. I hope that victory is right around the corner.

I would like to thank Bayhealth Medical's oncology nurses, the Delaware Breast Cancer Coalition, the Bringing Hope Home organization, all those who, helped, texted or called, prayed, or just said something nice or motivating on Facebook. It didn't go unnoticed or unappreciated.

www.ingramcontent.com/pod-product-compliance
Lightning Source LLC
Chambersburg PA
CBHW052126030426
42335CB00025B/3133